ANTI-PARKINSON COOKBOOK

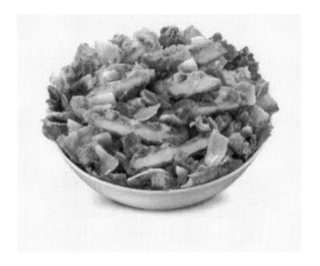

DR. JESSICA SMITH

TABLE OF CONTENT

INTRODUCTION

John was a middle-aged man who had been diagnosed with Parkinson's disease. He was devastated by the diagnosis and felt helpless in the face of his deteriorating health. He had tried all sorts of treatments and medications, but nothing seemed to help.

One day, John read an article online about how a specific diet could help reverse the symptoms of Parkinson's disease. He was ambiguous and wanted to give it a try.

John started by cutting out all processed foods, sugar, and dairy from his diet, and replacing them with whole grains, fresh fruits and vegetables, and lean proteins.

He also started taking supplements, including omega-3 fatty acids, which are thought to be beneficial for people with Parkinson's. Within a few months, John noticed a dramatic improvement in his symptoms.

He was able to move more easily, and his tremors were significantly reduced. He continued to follow the diet, and after a few more months, he was able to walk without assistance.

John was amazed by the results and began to share his story with other people who were living with Parkinson's. His story was a source of hope and inspiration for many.

John's story is a testament to the power of diet and nutrition in reversing Parkinson's disease. His success demonstrates that even the most devastating medical conditions can be improved through healthy lifestyle choices.

John's story is an inspiration to us all, and a reminder that we can take control of our health, even when faced with the most difficult of diagnoses.

John's story is proof that even when faced with the most challenging of medical conditions, we still have the power to take control of our health and our lives.

CHAPTER ONE

WHAT IS PARKINSON DISEASE?

Parkinson's disease (PD) is a progressive, degenerative neurological disorder that affects the central nervous system. It is characterized by a lack of coordination, trembling, rigidity, and difficulty walking.

The cause of Parkinson's is unknown, although some genetic factors may be involved. This disease has no cure but treatment may be use to reverse the disease

Parkinson's disease was first described by Dr. James Parkinson in 1817. He published an essay entitled "An Essay on the Shaking Palsy" in which he described the symptoms and characteristics of the disease.

Since then, it has been studied extensively and is now recognized as one of the most common neurological disorders.

The most common symptom of Parkinson's is tremor or shaking of the hands, arms, legs, jaw, or face. Other symptoms include slowness of movement, stiffness of the limbs or trunk, and impaired balance and coordination.

There may also be problems with speech, including slurring or difficulty forming words.

The exact cause of Parkinson's is still unknown, but it is believed to be related to a combination of genetic and environmental factors. Other factors may include

• Damage to the brain cells that produce a chemical messenger called dopamine

• Genetic mutations that affect the production of dopamine

• Exposure to environmental toxins

• Head trauma

• Certain medication

The symptoms of Parkinson's can vary from person to person, but the most common symptom is tremor. Other symptoms can include slowness of movement, stiffness of the limbs or trunk, impaired balance and coordination, and problems with speech. Treatment for Parkinson's aims to reduce the symptoms and improve quality of life.

Parkinson's disease is a complex condition that affects many aspects of a person's life. It is important to remember that it is a chronic condition and the symptoms can change over time.

With the right treatment and support, it is possible to live a full and active life with Parkinson's disease.

Finally, it is important to stay informed about research and advances in treatments for Parkinson's. Research is ongoing, and new treatments are being developed every day.

Staying informed about the latest developments can help you make informed decisions about your health and care.

Causes of Parkinson Disease

Parkinson disease (PD) is the second most common neurodegenerative disorder after Alzheimer's disease and affects approximately 1 million people in the United States.

The cause of PD is still largely unknown, and there is no single known cause. However, a number of factors, including genetics, environment, and lifestyle, are thought to contribute to the development of the condition.

Genetics: Mutations in certain genes are associated with an increased risk of PD. These include genes involved in the production of alpha-synuclein, a protein involved in synaptic function, and the genes encoding LRRK2, PINK1, and Parkin. Mutations in these genes can lead to an increased risk of developing PD.

Environment: Exposure to certain toxins, such as pesticides, may increase the risk of PD. Additionally, certain viruses, such as those causing the common cold, may also be associated with an increased risk of the disease.

Lifestyle: Smoking, depression, and stress can all increase the risk of PD, as can certain medications, such as antipsychotics.

Age: PD is more common in people over the age of 60.

Gender: Men are prone to PD than women

Although the exact cause of PD is still unknown, these factors may play a role in its development.

It is important to note that PD is not contagious and cannot be passed from one person to another.

Parkinson Disease sign and symptoms

Parkinson Disease (PD) is a progressive neurological disorder, caused by the loss of dopamine-producing neurons in the brain.

Motor symptoms include tremor, rigidity, slowed movement (bradykinesia), postural instability and impaired balance and coordination. Tremor is usually the most noticeable symptom and occurs as an involuntary rhythmic shaking in the hands, arms, legs, jaw, and face.

Rigidity is stiffness in the arms, legs, and trunk. Bradykinesia is the slowness of movement, and can make simple tasks like buttoning a shirt or writing difficult. Postural instability is the loss of balance and coordination, which makes it difficult to stand or walk without assistance.

Non-motor symptoms of PD include cognitive changes, such as difficulty with concentration and memory; sleep disturbances; depression; anxiety; and autonomic changes, such as difficulty with bladder control, constipation, and problems with temperature regulation.

People with PD may also experience pain, fatigue, and sensory changes, such as a decreased sense of touch and smell. PD can also cause vision problems and speech difficulties.

In addition to the physical symptoms of PD, people may also experience psychological issues, such as depression and anxiety. People with PD may also experience social challenges, such as difficulty communicating and interacting with others.

PD is commonly diagnosed in people over the age of 50, however, it can occur in younger people as well. PD is a chronic and progressive disorder, meaning that symptoms can get worse over time. There is currently no cure for PD, but medications, surgery, and physical and occupational therapy can help manage symptoms.

It is important to talk to a doctor if you or a loved one is experiencing any of the signs and symptoms of Parkinson Disease.

Early diagnosis and treatment can help improve quality of life and slow the progression of the disease.

Treatment of Parkinson disease

Medication: The mainstay of treatment for Parkinson's disease is medication.

Commonly prescribed drugs include Levodopa, which is the most effective drug for reducing the symptoms, and dopamine agonists, which help to replicate the effects of dopamine in the body. Other medications used to treat Parkinson's disease include anticholinergics, MAO-B inhibitors, and COMT inhibitors

Surgery: In some cases, surgery may be recommended to help control the symptoms of Parkinson's disease. Deep brain stimulation is a procedure that involves implanting electrodes in the brain to stimulate specific areas affected by the disease. It is used to reduce tremor, stiffness, and other symptoms.

Lifestyle Changes: Making lifestyle changes can help to reduce the severity of symptoms and improve quality of life. These may include exercise, eating a healthy diet, avoiding stress and caffeine, and taking part in social activities

Therapy: Physical and occupational therapies can help to improve mobility and reduce the risk of falls. Speech therapy can be used to improve mode of communication or communication skills. Cognitive behavioral therapy can help to improve mood and reduce anxiety

Prevention of Parkinson disease

Till date, there is no specific way or guide to prevent Parkinson's disease. However, there are some lifestyle changes that may help to reduce the risk:

• Eating a healthy diet: Eating a diet that is rich in fruits and vegetables and low in saturated fats can help to reduce the risk of developing Parkinson's disease.

• Exercising regularly: Regular exercise can help to maintain muscle strength and reduce the risk of chronic diseases, such as Parkinson's disease.

• Avoiding environmental toxins: Avoiding exposure to environmental toxins, such as pesticides, herbicides, and heavy metals, may help to reduce the risk of developing Parkinson's disease.

Diagnosis of Parkinson disease

Parkinson's disease is typically diagnosed by a neurologist. A physical exam and a review of medical history are used to diagnose the condition. Other tests, such as a brain scan or blood test, may be used to confirm the diagnosis.

In some cases, a trial of medication may be recommended to help the doctor determine if the symptoms are due to Parkinson's disease.

As soon as the diagnosis is carried out, treatment can begin. Treatment plans will vary depending on the individual, but the goal is to reduce symptoms and improve quality of life.

Parkinson disease foods to eat and avoid

PD is a neurological condition that progresses and affects movement and coordination in the human body. It is caused by the loss of dopamine-producing nerve cells in the brain. While there is no cure for Parkinson's disease, eating a balanced diet can help manage symptoms and improve quality of life.

Foods to Eat

A healthy diet for people with Parkinson's disease should include plenty of fruits, vegetables, whole grains, legumes, lean proteins, and healthy fats.

Fruits and Vegetables: Fruits and vegetables are high in antioxidants and other nutrients that can help protect against cell damage and inflammation. Also, they are low in calories, so they can help with weight management.

Whole Grains: Whole grains are packed with fiber, vitamins, and minerals, making them a great choice for people with Parkinson's. Examples of whole grains are oats, brown rice, quinoa, and barley.

Legumes: Legumes, such as beans, lentils, and peas, are high in protein, fiber, and essential vitamins and minerals. They are also low in fat and contain a variety of antioxidants.

Lean Proteins: Lean proteins, such as fish, chicken, and turkey, are an important part of a healthy diet. They provide essential amino acids and are low in saturated fat.

Healthy Fats: Healthy fats, such as olive oil, avocados, and nuts, are important for brain health and can help manage inflammation.

Foods to Avoid

In addition to eating a balanced diet, it is important to limit or avoid certain foods that can worsen Parkinson's disease symptoms. These include:

Processed Foods: Processed foods are often high in sugar, sodium, and unhealthy fats, which can increase inflammation and worsen Parkinson's symptoms.

Sugary Foods and Drinks: Too much sugar can increase inflammation and disrupt blood sugar levels. It is best to limit sugary foods and drinks, such as candy, soda, and other sweetened beverages.

Fried Foods: Fried foods are high in fat and calories and can worsen inflammation. It is best to limit or avoid fried foods, such as French fries and fried chicken.

Alcohol: Alcohol can worsen tremors, reduce coordination, and disrupt sleep. It is best to limit or avoid alcohol if you have Parkinson's disease.

Caffeine: Caffeine can worsen tremors and disrupt sleep. It is best to limit or avoid caffeine if you have Parkinson's disease.

By eating a balanced diet and avoiding certain foods, people with Parkinson's disease can help manage their symptoms and improve their quality of life. If you have questions about what to eat, talk to your doctor or a registered dietitian.

CHAPTER TWO

The role of diet and exercise in reversing Parkinson disease

Exercise has been found to be a beneficial treatment for Parkinson's disease. It has been found to help improve balance, coordination, posture, walking speed, and overall physical functioning.

Exercise can also help reduce fatigue, improve quality of life, and even slow the progression of the disease. Exercise can also help reduce symptoms of depression, which is common in Parkinson's sufferers.

Regular exercise can help reduce the risk of falls and improve overall physical health, which can help reduce the risk of secondary complications associated with the disease. Exercise can also help improve cognitive functioning and can help reduce the risk of dementia.

Exercise has been found to help the body utilize dopamine more effectively, which can help improve symptoms of the disease.

Finally, exercise has been found to help reduce pain and stiffness in the muscles, which can help improve movement.

Overall, exercise has been found to be a beneficial treatment for Parkinson's disease. It can help improve physical and cognitive functioning, reduce symptoms of depression, and reduce the risk of secondary complications.

It can also help the body utilize dopamine more effectively, reduce pain and stiffness, and improve movement. Regular exercise can help improve the quality of life of those living with Parkinson's disease.

Although exercise is beneficial for Parkinson's disease sufferers, it should not be done without medical supervision. Exercise should be tailored to the individual's needs and abilities and should be done under the guidance of a qualified medical professional.

Furthermore, it is important to remember that exercise is just one element of a comprehensive treatment plan for Parkinson's disease. Other treatments such as medications, lifestyle changes, and physical and occupational therapy may be necessary in order to achieve the best possible outcome.

In conclusion, exercise is an important part of reversing Parkinson's disease. It can help improve physical and cognitive functioning, reduce symptoms of depression, and reduce the risk of secondary complications.

Furthermore, it can help the body utilize dopamine more effectively, reduce pain and stiffness, and improve movement. Exercise should be done under the supervision of a qualified medical professional and should be part of a comprehensive treatment plan in order to achieve the best possible outcome.

Parkinson disease diet and exercise are important factors in managing symptoms and overall health. Diet and exercise can help improve mobility, reduce fatigue, and improve quality of life.

Eating a balanced diet, with plenty of fresh fruits, vegetables, lean proteins, and healthy fats can help provide the nutrition needed to manage the symptoms of Parkinson's disease.

Additionally, regular exercise can help improve balance, flexibility, and strength, and reduce the risk of falls. When it comes to diet, the main goal is to maintain a healthy weight, as being overweight or obese can have a negative impact on the progression of the disease. It's important to get enough protein, carbohydrates, and fat in the diet, and to limit processed foods, sugar, and saturated fat.

Eating a variety of foods can help ensure that all essential nutrients are consumed. Some foods that may be beneficial for people with Parkinson's disease include:

• Fish, poultry, and legumes

• Fruits and vegetables such as apples, oranges, spinach, and broccoli

• Whole grains such as oats, quinoa, and brown rice

•Some healthy calories from sources such as nuts, seeds, avocados, and olive oil

• Low-fat dairy products

In addition to eating a balanced diet, exercise is important for people with Parkinson's disease. Exercise can help improve mobility, reduce fatigue, and improve overall quality of life. It can also help to maintain muscle strength, reduce stress, and improve balance. In addition, some kinds of exercises that may help and be beneficial include:

- Weight training to build muscle strength

- Walking or running for aerobic exercise

- Yoga exercises or tai chi for free movement or body flexibility and balance

- Swimming or cycling for cardiovascular fitness

- Balance or stability exercises such as walking heel to toe

Eating a healthy diet and engaging in regular exercise can be beneficial for people with Parkinson's disease. It's important to discuss any changes to diet and exercise with a healthcare provider before making any changes.

Additionally, it's important to listen to the body and rest when needed. With the right diet and exercise plan, people with Parkinson's disease can improve their overall health and well-being.

In conclusion, once you have tried living a healthy life, eat good diet and exercise regularly and the disease still persist, it is best to visit your doctor and discuss the issue.

Your doctor may suggest that you take medications that can help alleviate the symptoms of the condition or refer you to a specialist for further evaluation and treatment.

CHAPTER THREE

ANTI-PARKINSON DISEASE RECIPES

1. Fruit Smoothie:

Ingredients:

-2 cups of frozen fruit of your choice (strawberries, blueberries, etc.)

-1 cup of unsweetened almond milk

-1 tablespoon of flaxseed

-1 tablespoon of honey

Instructions:

-Put all ingredients in a blender, mix and blend until the fruits are smooth and suitable for consumption

-Enjoy your delicious and nutritious smoothie!

2. Spinach Quinoa Salad:

Ingredients:

-1 cup cooked quinoa

-2 cups spinach, chopped

-1/2 cup cherry tomatoes, halved

-2 tablespoons of lemon juice

-1 tablespoon of olive oil

-Salt and pepper, to taste

Instructions:

-In a medium bowl, combine cooked quinoa, spinach, and cherry tomatoes.

-Lemon juice and olive oil, in a separate bowl mixed together

-Pour the lemon juice mixture over the quinoa mixture and toss to combine.

-Season with salt and pepper, to taste.

-Serve and enjoy!

3. Salmon with Asparagus:

Ingredients:

-2 salmon fillets

-1 teaspoon of garlic powder

-1 teaspoon of onion powder

-1 teaspoon of paprika

-1/2 teaspoon of salt

-1/4 teaspoon of black pepper

-2 tablespoons of butter

-1 bunch of asparagus

Instructions:

-Preheat oven to 350°F.

-combine garlic powder, onion powder, paprika, salt & black pepper in a small plate

- Over the salmon fillets, mix with the ingredients

-Heat the butter to melt in a big bowl over medium temperature

-Add salmon fillets and cook until lightly browned, about 3 minutes per side.

-Transfer the salmon to a baking dish.

-Add asparagus to the same skillet and cook until lightly browned, about 3 minutes.

-Transfer the asparagus to the baking dish with the salmon.

-Bake in preheated oven for 10–12 minutes, or until the salmon is cooked through and the asparagus is tender.

-Serve and enjoy!

4. Lentil Soup:

Ingredients:

-1 tablespoon of olive oil

-1 onion, diced

-2 cloves of garlic, minced

-2 cups of lentils, rinsed and drained

-4 cups of vegetable broth

-1 teaspoon of dried oregano

-1 teaspoon of dried thyme

-1 teaspoon of smoked paprika

-1/2 teaspoon of salt

-1/4 teaspoon of pepper

Instructions:

-In a big pot, preheat the olive oil over a medium temperature.

-About 5 minutes, add onion and garlic then cook.

-Add lentils, vegetable broth, oregano, thyme, smoked paprika, salt, and pepper.

-Bring to a boil, reduce heat to low, and simmer for 25–30 minutes, or until the lentils are tender.

-Preferably use an immersion blender and blend the soup until desired.

-Serve and enjoy!

5. Vegetable Stir Fry:

Ingredients:

-1 tablespoon of olive oil

-1 onion, diced

-2 cloves of garlic, minced

-1 bell pepper, diced

-1 cup of broccoli florets

-1 cup of sliced mushrooms

-1/4 cup of vegetable broth

-1/2 teaspoon of garlic powder

-1/2 teaspoon of onion powder

-1/2 teaspoon of dried oregano

-1/2 teaspoon of dried thyme

-Salt and pepper, to taste

Instructions:

-Over medium temperature in a big bowl, heat the oil

-Cook and allow to soft for about 5 minutes then add onion and garlic

-Add bell pepper, broccoli, mushrooms, vegetable broth, garlic powder, onion powder, oregano, and thyme.

-Cook vegetables for 10 minutes until they are soft.

-Season with salt and pepper, to taste.

-Serve and enjoy!

6. Sweet Potato and Avocado Mash:

Ingredients:

- Peel & diced 2 big sweet potatoes

- 1 ripe avocado, pitted and peeled

- 2 tablespoons olive oil

- 1 teaspoon ground turmeric

- Salt and pepper to taste

Instructions:

1. Preheat oven to 400 degrees F.

2. Place the diced sweet potatoes on a baking sheet and drizzle with olive oil.

3. Allow and bake for more than 20 minutes until potatoes are soft

4. Place the avocado, sweet potatoes, olive oil, turmeric, salt and pepper in a food processor and blend until smooth.

5. Serve warm or chilled.

7. Coconut Curry Soup:

Ingredients:

- 2 tablespoons olive oil

- 1 onion, diced

- 2 cloves garlic, minced

- 2 teaspoons curry powder

- 1 teaspoon ground turmeric

- 1 can coconut milk

- 2 cups vegetable broth

- 2 cups chopped kale

- 1 carrot, diced

- 2 tablespoons fresh parsley, chopped

- Salt and pepper to taste

Instructions:

1. In a big pot, preheat over a medium temperature

2. About 5 minutes or more, add onion and garlic and cook until tender

3. Stir in the curry powder and turmeric and cook for 1 minute.

4. Add the coconut milk and vegetable broth and bring to a simmer.

5. Add the kale, carrot, and parsley and simmer for 10 minutes.

6. Mix or dice with salt and pepper

7. Serve warm.

8. Salmon and Asparagus:

Ingredients:

- 4 (4-ounce) salmon fillets

- 2 tablespoons olive oil

- Salt and pepper to taste

- 1/2-pound asparagus, trimmed

- 2 tablespoons lemon juice

- 2 tablespoons fresh dill, chopped

Instructions:

1. Preheat oven to 400 degrees F.

2. Place the salmon fillets on a baking sheet and brush with olive oil.

3. Use salt and pepper for seasoning and to taste nice.

4. Bake for 10 minutes or until salmon is cooked through.

5. Meanwhile, steam the asparagus for 8 minutes or until tender.

6. Toss with lemon juice, dill, salt and pepper to taste.

7. Serve with the salmon.

9. Quinoa Pilaf:

Ingredients:

- 1 tablespoon olive oil

- 1 onion, diced

- 2 cloves garlic, minced

- 1 cup quinoa, rinsed

- 2 cups vegetable broth

- 1 cup diced bell pepper

- 1/2 cup chopped walnuts

- 2 tablespoons fresh parsley, chopped

- Salt and pepper to taste

Instructions:

1. In a big pot, preheat the oil over a medium temperature

2. About 5 minutes, add onion and garlic then cook.

3. Stir in the quinoa and vegetable broth and bring to a simmer.

4. Reduce heat to low and simmer, covered, for 15 minutes or until quinoa is tender.

5. Stir in the bell pepper and walnuts and cook for 5 minutes.

6. Stir in the parsley, salt and pepper to taste.

7. Serve warm.

10. Blueberry Smoothie:

Ingredients:

- 1 cup frozen blueberries

- 1/2 banana

- 1/2 cup plain Greek yogurt

- 1/4 cup almond milk

- 2 tablespoons chia seeds

Instructions:

1. Put all the fruits ingredients in a blender and blend accordingly till smooth then

2. Pour into

11. Oatmeal and Flaxseed Breakfast Bowl:

Ingredients:

-1/2 cup rolled oats

-1/4 cup ground flaxseed

-1/2 cup low-fat milk

-1 teaspoon honey

-1/4 teaspoon ground cinnamon

-1/4 cup fresh blueberries

Instructions:

1. Boil one cup of water in a medium saucepan

2. Add the oats and reduce the heat to a simmer. Cook for 5 minutes, stirring occasionally.

3. Add the flaxseed, milk, honey, and cinnamon. Cook for another 5 minutes.

4. Divide into different bowls and after removed from the heated temperature.

5. Top with the blueberries and serve.

12. Broccoli and Avocado Salad:

Ingredients:

-2 cups broccoli florets

-1/2 avocado, diced

-1/4 cup diced red onion

-1/4 cup diced cucumber

-1/4 cup finely chopped parsley

-2 tablespoons olive oil

-2 tablespoons lemon juice

-1/4 teaspoon sea salt

Instructions:

1. Place the broccoli florets in a steamer basket over a pot of boiling water. Cover and steam for 5 minutes.

2. In a large bowl, combine the avocado, red onion, cucumber, and parsley.

3. In a small bowl, whisk together the olive oil, lemon juice, and sea salt.

4. Pour the dressing over the salad and toss to coat.

5. Add the steamed broccoli and toss again. Serve.

13. Spinach and Mushroom Quinoa:

Ingredients:

-1 cup quinoa, rinsed

-2 cups vegetable broth

-1 tablespoon olive oil

-1 cup sliced mushrooms

-1 cup chopped spinach

-1/4 teaspoon garlic powder

-1/4 teaspoon onion powder

-1/4 teaspoon black pepper

Instructions:

1. Bring the quinoa and veggies broth to a boil In a medium saucepan, bring down the heat temperature and simmer for 15 minutes, or until the quinoa is cooked.

2. In a big pot, preheat the oil over a medium temperature

3. 3 minutes interval, add mushroom and saute

4. Add the spinach, garlic powder, onion powder, and black pepper. Cook for another 2 minutes.

5. Add the cooked quinoa to the skillet and stir to combine. Cook for another 2 minutes. Serve.

14. Lentil and Kale Soup:

Ingredients:

-1 tablespoon olive oil

-1 onion, diced

-1 carrot, diced

-1 celery stalk, diced

-2 cloves garlic, minced

-1 teaspoon ground cumin

-1 teaspoon dried oregano

-1/2 teaspoon paprika

-1/4 teaspoon ground black pepper

-4 cups vegetable broth

-1 cup green lentils, rinsed

-1 cup chopped kale

Instructions:

1. In a big pot, preheat the oil over a medium temperature

2. Add the onion, carrot, celery, and garlic. Cook for 5 minutes, stirring occasionally.

3. Add the cumin, oregano, paprika, and black pepper. Cook for another minute.

4. Add the vegetable broth, lentils, and kale.

5. Bring to a boil, reduce heat and simmer for 30 minutes, or until the lentils are tender. Serve.

15. Baked Salmon with Asparagus

Ingredients:

-2 (6-ounce) salmon fillets

-1/2 teaspoon garlic powder

-1/2 teaspoon onion powder

-1/2 teaspoon paprika

-1/4 teaspoon ground black pepper

-1/4 teaspoon sea salt

-1 tablespoon olive oil

-1 bunch asparagus, trimmed

Instructions:

1. Heat oven to 400 degrees Fahrenheit.

2. Put the salmon fillets on a baking tray lined with parchment paper.

3. In a small bowl, mix together the garlic powder, onion powder, paprika, black pepper, and sea salt. Rub the mixture over the salmon.

4. Drizzle the olive oil over the salmon and asparagus.

5. Bake for 12-15 minutes, or until the salmon is cooked through. Serve.

16. Turmeric and Ginger Tea

Ingredients:

-1 teaspoon of ground turmeric

-1 teaspoon of ground ginger

-2 cups of water

Instructions:

-Put all the boiled water to a small saucepan.

-Add the turmeric and ginger and reduce the heat to low.

-Simmer for 10 minutes and strain the mixture.

-Serve warm or cold.

17. Broccoli Soup

Ingredients:

-4 cups of broccoli, finely chopped

-1 onion, diced

-1 clove of garlic, minced

-2 tablespoons of olive oil

-2 cups of vegetable stock

-1 teaspoon of turmeric

-Salt and pepper to taste

Instructions:

-In a big saucepan, preheat the olive oil over a medium temperature

-Furthermore, add in onion and garlic and cook until it becomes soft.

-In a short while add the broccoli and cook

-Add the veggies stock and put to a simmer.

-Garnish/Season with salt and pepper then add some turmeric of your taste

-Simmer until the broccoli is tender.

-Blend the soup until smooth.

-Serve warm.

18. Baked Fish with Turmeric and Ginger

Ingredients:

-4 fish fillets

-2 tablespoons of olive oil

-2 teaspoons of ground turmeric

-2 teaspoons of ground ginger

-1 teaspoon of garlic powder

-Salt and pepper to taste

Instructions:

-Preheat the oven to 350 degrees F.

-Line a baking sheet with parchment paper.

-In a baking sheet pan and put the fish fillets

-Drizzle the olive oil over the fish.

-Sprinkle the turmeric, ginger, garlic powder, salt, and pepper over the fish.

-Bake in a heated oven for 15-20 minutes max or until the fish is cooked to your taste

-Serve warm.

19. Avocado and Turmeric Smoothie

Ingredients:

-1 ripe avocado

-1/2 cup of almond milk

-1 tablespoon of honey

-1 teaspoon of ground turmeric

-1/2 teaspoon of ground ginger

Instructions:

-Combine all ingredients in a blender.

-Blend until smooth.

-Serve chilled.

20. Turmeric-Ginger Oatmeal

Ingredients:

-1 cup of old-fashioned oats

-2 cups of water

-1 teaspoon of ground turmeric

-1 teaspoon of ground ginger

-1/4 cup of diced fresh fruit

-1 tablespoon of honey

Instructions:

-Bring the water and allow to boil in a medium temperature saucepan.

-In addition, reduce to low medium temperature hear and add the oats

-Stir in the turmeric and ginger and cook for 5 minutes.

-Remove from heat and stir in the diced fruit and honey.

-Serve warm.

21. Oats, Berries and Walnuts Smoothie

Ingredients:

- 1/2 cup of oats

- 1/2 cup of frozen berries

- 1/4 cup of walnuts

- 1 cup of almond milk

- 1 tablespoon of honey

Instructions:

- Place oats, berries, and walnuts into a blender.

- Pour almond milk into the blender.

- Blend until all ingredients are mixed together.

- Add honey and blend again.

- Serve cold or at room temperature.

22. Apple and Cinnamon Yogurt Bowl

Ingredients:

- 1 apple, chopped

- 1/2 teaspoon of ground cinnamon

- 1 cup of plain yogurt

- 1 tablespoon of honey

Instructions:

- In a big bowl or plate, put the sliced or chopped apple.

- Sprinkle with ground cinnamon.

- Pour in the yogurt and stir.

- Add honey and stir again.

- Serve cold or at room temperature.

23. Roasted Sweet Potato and Broccoli Bowl

Ingredients:

- 1 sweet potato, cubed

- 1 big head of green broccoli, cut into florets

- 1 tablespoon of olive oil

- Salt and pepper to taste

Instructions:

- Preheat oven to 400°F.

- Place cubed sweet potatoes and broccoli florets on a baking sheet.

- Garnish with salt and pepper to taste sweet and Drizzle with olive oil and seasoning

- Dry or Roast for about 20 minutes or more until veggies are tender or soft.

- Place in a bowl and serve.

24. Lentil and Spinach Soup

Ingredients:

- 1 tablespoon of olive oil

- 1 onion, chopped

- 2 cloves of garlic, minced

- 1 cup of dried lentils

- 4 cups of vegetable broth

- 2 cups of spinach, chopped

- Salt and pepper to taste

Instructions:

- In a big pot, preheat the olive oil over a medium temperature

- Allow too soft for at least 5 minutes then add onion, garlic and saute.

- Bring boiled, add lentils and veggies broth.

- Bring down the heat and allow cool for 15 minutes.

- Add some more spinach to make it much and cool for 5 more minutes max.

- Garnish, season everything them with salt and pepper to taste nice.

- Serve hot.

25. Quinoa and Kale Salad

Ingredients:

- 1 cup of cooked quinoa

- 2 cups of kale, chopped

- 1/4 cup of sunflower seeds

- 1/4 cup of cranberries

- 2 tablespoons of olive oil

- 2 tablespoons of apple cider vinegar

- Salt and pepper to taste

Instructions:

- Place cooked quinoa, kale, sunflower seeds, and cranberries in a large bowl.

-Mix together olive oil, apple cider vinegar, salt and pepper in a small bowl or plate

- Mixed salad and pour the dressings till everything is combined.

- Serve cold or at room temperature.

26. Broccoli and Tofu Stir-Fry

Ingredients:

- 2 tablespoons of olive oil

- 1/2 cup of diced onions

- 2 cloves of minced garlic

-1 big head of green broccoli, cut into florets

- 1/2 block of extra-firm tofu, cubed

- 1 teaspoon of sesame oil

- 2 tablespoons of low-sodium soy sauce

Instructions:

1. In a big pot, preheat the olive oil over a medium temperature

2. Add the onions and garlic and cook until softened, about 5 minutes.

3. Add the broccoli and tofu and cook until the broccoli is tender, about 8 minutes.

4. Add the sesame oil and soy sauce and stir to combine.

5. Serve over cooked brown rice or quinoa.

27. Quinoa Power Bowl

Ingredients:

- 1 cup of quinoa

- 1 tablespoon of olive oil

- 2 cloves of minced garlic

- 1/2 teaspoon of ground turmeric

- 1/2 teaspoon of ground cumin

- 1/2 teaspoon of ground coriander

- 1/4 teaspoon of ground ginger

- 1/4 teaspoon of ground cardamom

- 1 chickpeas can, drained, rinsed or washed in a bowl

- 1 cup of diced bell peppers

- 1/2 cup of diced carrots

- 1/2 cup of diced zucchini

- 1/2 cup of diced tomatoes

- 2 tablespoons of lemon juice

- 2 tablespoons of chopped fresh parsley

Instructions:

1. Place the quinoa in a medium saucepan and add 2 cups of water. Bring the water to a boil, reduce the heat to low, and simmer for 15 minutes, or until the quinoa is cooked.

2. In a big pot, preheat the olive oil over a medium temperature and add the garlic and cook for 1 minute.

3. Add the turmeric, cumin, coriander, ginger, and cardamom and stir to combine.

4. Add the chickpeas, bell peppers, carrots, zucchini, and tomatoes and cook for 5 minutes, or until the vegetables are tender.

5. Add the cooked quinoa to the skillet and stir to combine.

6. Remove from the heat and stir in the lemon juice and parsley.

7. Serve warm.

28. Lentil and Spinach Soup

Ingredients:

- 2 tablespoons of olive oil

- 1/2 cup of diced onions

- 2 cloves of minced garlic

- 1 teaspoon of ground cumin

- 1 teaspoon of ground coriander

- 1/2 teaspoon of ground turmeric

- 1 cup of dried lentils

- 4 cups of vegetable broth

- 1 can of diced tomatoes

- 2 cups of packed spinach

- Salt and pepper to taste

Instructions:

1. In a big pot, preheat the olive oil over a medium temperature

2. Add the onions and garlic and cook until softened, about 5 minutes.

3. Add the cumin, coriander, and turmeric and stir to combine.

4. Add the lentils and vegetable broth and bring to a boil.

5. Reduce the heat to low and simmer for 15 minutes, or until the lentils are tender.

6. Add the tomatoes and spinach and cook for 5 minutes, or until the spinach is wilted.

7. Garnish/Season with salt and pepper to taste nicely for you.

8. Serve warm.

29. Zucchini Noodles with Avocado Sauce

Ingredients:

- 2 tablespoons of olive oil

- 2 cloves of minced garlic

- 2 zucchini, spiralized into noodles

- 1/2 cup of chopped fresh basil

- 1/4 teaspoon of red pepper flakes

- 1/4 cup of diced tomatoes

- 1 avocado

- 2 tablespoons of lemon juice

- 2 tablespoons of olive oil

- Salt and pepper to taste

Instructions:

1. In a big pot, preheat the olive oil over a medium temperature

2. Add garlic and cook for not more than 1 minute.

3. Add the zucchini noodles, basil, and red pepper flakes and cook for 5 minutes, or until the noodles are tender.

4. In a blender, combine the avocado, lemon juice, and olive oil and blend until smooth.

5. Add the diced tomatoes to the skillet and cook for an additional 2 minutes.

6. Pour the avocado sauce over the noodles and stir to combine.

7. Garnish or Season with salt and pepper to taste nicely.

8. Serve warm.

30. Lentil and Kale Salad

Ingredients:

- 1 cup of dried lentils

- 2 tablespoons of olive oil

- 1/2 teaspoon of ground cumin

- 1/4 teaspoon of ground coriander

- 1/4 teaspoon of ground turmeric

- 1/4 teaspoon of ground ginger

- 2 cloves of minced garlic

- 2 cups of chopped kale

- 1/4 cup of diced red onion

- 1/4 cup of diced cucumber

- 2 tablespoons of lemon juice

- 2 tablespoons of chopped fresh parsley

- Salt and pepper to taste

Instructions:

1. Place the lentils in a medium saucepan and add 2 cups of water. Bring the water to a boil, reduce the heat to low, and simmer for 15 minutes, or until the lentils are tender.

2. In a big pot, preheat the olive oil over a medium temperature

3. Add the cumin, coriander, turmeric, ginger, and garlic and cook for 1 minute.

4. Add the kale and cook for 5 minutes, or until the kale is wilted.

5. In a large bowl, combine the cooked lentils, kale, red onion, cucumber, lemon juice, and parsley.

6. Garnish or Season with salt and pepper to taste nicely.

7. Serve warm or cold.

31. Banana Blueberry Oatmeal Smoothie

Ingredients:

- 1 ripe banana

- 1/2 cup plain Greek yogurt

- 1/2 cup frozen blueberries

- 1/2 cup rolled oats

- 1/2 cup almond milk

- 1 teaspoon honey

Instructions:

1. Place the banana, yogurt, blueberries, oats, almond milk, and honey in a blender.

2. Blend until smooth.

3. Serve chilled.

32. Avocado Toast with Hemp Seeds

Ingredients:

- 2 slices whole grain bread

- 1 ripe avocado

- 2 tablespoons hemp seeds

- 1/4 teaspoon garlic powder

- 1/4 teaspoon sea salt

Instructions:

1. Toast the bread until golden brown.

2. Mash the avocado in a bowl and season with garlic powder and sea salt.

3. Spread or place the mashed or diced avocado on the toast.

4. Sprinkle with hemp seeds.

5. Serve.

33. Roasted Chickpeas

Ingredients:

- 1 (15-ounce) can chickpeas, drained and rinsed or washed

- 2 tablespoons olive oil

- 1 teaspoon garlic powder

- 1 teaspoon paprika

- 1/2 teaspoon sea salt

Instructions:

1. Preheat the oven to 375°F.

2. Place a baking sheet with parchment paper.

3. Place the chickpeas on the baking sheet and drizzle with olive oil.

4. Sprinkle with garlic powder, paprika, and sea salt.

5. Toss to coat.

6. Roast for 30 minutes, stirring once halfway through.

7. Serve warm.

34. Apple and Almond Butter Snack

Ingredients:

- 1 apple, sliced

- 2 tablespoons almond butter

- 1 teaspoon chia seeds

- 1/2 teaspoon ground cinnamon

Instructions:

1. Lay the apple slices on a plate.

2. Spread the almond butter evenly over the apple slices.

3. Sprinkle with chia seeds and cinnamon.

4. Serve.

35. Cucumber Hummus Bites

Ingredients:

- 1 cucumber, sliced

- 1/4 cup hummus

- 2 tablespoons chopped fresh parsley

Instructions:

1. Place the cucumber slices on a plate.

2. Spread the hummus on the cucumber slices.

3. Sprinkle with parsley.

4. Serve.

36. Banana and Peanut Butter Smoothie:

Ingredients:

- 2 Bananas

- 2 tablespoons of creamy peanut butter

- 1 cup of almond milk

- 1 teaspoon of honey

Instructions:

- Place the bananas, peanut butter, almond milk, and honey into a blender.

- Blend until smooth.

- Pour into a glass and enjoy!

37. Apple and Walnut Oatmeal:

Ingredients:

- 1/2 cup of rolled oats

- 1/2 cup of almond milk

- 1 diced apple

- 2 tablespoons of chopped walnuts

- A pinch of cinnamon

Instructions:

- Place the oats and almond milk in a saucepan and bring to a boil.

- Bring the temperature (heat) down and simmer for 3 minutes.

- Add the diced apple, walnuts, and cinnamon and stir to combine.

- Cook for a further 5 minutes.

- Serve warm and enjoy!

38. Quinoa and Avocado Salad:

Ingredients:

- 1/2 cup of cooked quinoa

- 1 diced avocado

- 1/2 cup of cherry tomatoes, halved

- 2 tablespoons of olive oil

- Juice of 1/2 a lemon

- Salt and pepper to taste

Instructions:

- Place the cooked quinoa, avocado, and tomatoes in a bowl.

- Drizzle the olive oil and lemon juice over the top and season with salt and pepper.

- Toss to combine and serve.

39. Blueberry and Yogurt Parfait:

Ingredients:

- 1 cup of plain Greek yogurt

- 1/2 cup of blueberries

- 2 tablespoons of sliced almonds

- 2 tablespoons of honey

Instructions:

- Place the yogurt in a bowl and top with the blueberries, almonds, and honey.

- Mix together and enjoy!

40. Tomato and Spinach Soup

Ingredients:

-2 tablespoons olive oil

-1 onion, chopped

-2 cloves garlic, minced

-3 tomatoes, peeled and chopped

-3 cups chicken or vegetable broth

-1/4 teaspoon ground black pepper

-1/4 teaspoon dried oregano

-2 cups fresh spinach leaves, chopped

-1/4 cup heavy cream (optional)

Instructions:

1. In a big pot, preheat the olive oil over a medium temperature

2. Add the onion and garlic and sauté for 3-4 minutes, until the onion is soft and translucent.

3. Add the tomatoes, broth, pepper, and oregano. Boil all the mixture and then reduce the heat to medium temperature and simmer for 10 minutes.

4. Stir in the spinach and simmer for an additional 5 minutes.

5. Remove the pot from the heat and let cool for 5 minutes.

6. Pour the soup in a blender and blend until smooth throughout.

7. Return the soup to the pot and stir in the heavy cream, if desired.

8. Reheat the soup over low heat and serve.

41. Peach and Coconut Smoothie:

Ingredients:

-1 cup frozen peaches

-1/2 cup coconut milk

-1/4 cup plain Greek yogurt

-1 tablespoon honey

-1/2 teaspoon ground cinnamon

Instructions:

1. Put all ingredients in a blender and blend smooth till it is suitable for drinking

2. Pour into a glass and enjoy.

42. Mixed Berry Smoothie:

Ingredients:

-1 cup strawberries

-1/2 cup blueberries

-1/2 cup raspberries

-1/2 cup coconut milk

-1 tablespoon honey

-1/2 teaspoon ground ginger

Instructions:

1. Put all ingredients in a blender and blend smooth till it is suitable for drinking

2. Pour into a glass and enjoy.

43. Orange-Mango Smoothie:

Ingredients:

-1 cup orange juice

-1 cup frozen mango chunks

-1/2 cup plain Greek yogurt

-1 tablespoon honey

-1/2 teaspoon ground turmeric

Instructions:

1. Put all ingredients in a blender and blend smooth till it is suitable for drinking

2. Pour into a glass and enjoy.

44. Green Tea and Mint Smoothie:

Ingredients:

-1 cup brewed green tea

-1/2 cup frozen spinach

-1/2 cup plain Greek yogurt

-1 tablespoon honey

-1/2 teaspoon mint extract

Instructions:

1. Put all ingredients in a blender and blend smooth till it is suitable for drinking

2. Pour into a glass and enjoy.

45. Pineapple-Lime Smoothie:

Ingredients:

-1 cup pineapple juice

-1/2 cup frozen pineapple chunks

-1/2 cup plain Greek yogurt

-1 tablespoon honey

-1/2 teaspoon lime zest

Instructions:

1. Put all ingredients in a blender and blend smooth till it is suitable for drinking

2. Pour into a glass and enjoy.

46. Banana-Almond Smoothie:

Ingredients:

-1 cup banana slices

-1/2 cup almond milk

-1/2 cup plain Greek yogurt

-1 tablespoon honey

-1/2 teaspoon ground cinnamon

Instructions:

1. Put all ingredients in a blender and blend smooth till it is suitable for drinking

2. Pour into a glass and enjoy.

47. Mango-Papaya Smoothie:

Ingredients:

-1 cup mango chunks

-1/2 cup papaya chunks

-1/2 cup coconut milk

-1 tablespoon honey

-1/2 teaspoon ground ginger

Instructions:

1. Put all ingredients in a blender and blend smooth till it is suitable for drinking

2. Pour into a glass and enjoy.

48. Strawberry-Cocoa Smoothie:

Ingredients:

-1 cup frozen strawberries

-1/2 cup almond milk

-1/2 cup plain Greek yogurt

-1 tablespoon honey

-1/2 teaspoon cocoa powder

Instructions:

1. Put all ingredients in a blender and blend smooth till it is suitable for drinking

2. Pour into a glass and enjoy.

49. Blueberry-Coconut Smoothie:

Ingredients:

-1 cup frozen blueberries

-1/2 cup coconut milk

-1/2 cup plain Greek yogurt

-1 tablespoon honey

-1/2 teaspoon ground cardamom

Instructions:

1. Put all ingredients in a blender and blend smooth till it is suitable for drinking.

2. Pour into a glass and enjoy.

50. Banana-Cherry Smoothie:

Ingredients:

-1 cup banana slices

-1/2 cup frozen cherries

-1/2 cup plain Greek yogurt

-1 tablespoon honey

-1/2 teaspoon ground nutmeg

Instructions:

1. Put all ingredients in a blender and blend smooth till it is suitable for drinking

2. Pour into a glass and enjoy.

51. Melon-Coconut Smoothie:

Ingredients:

-1 cup diced cantaloupe

-1/2 cup coconut milk

-1/2 cup plain Greek yogurt

-1 tablespoon honey

-1/2 teaspoon ground ginger

Instructions:

1. Put all ingredients in a blender and blend smooth till it is suitable for drinking.

2. Pour into a glass and enjoy.

52. Apple-Cinnamon Smoothie:

Ingredients:

-1 cup diced apples

-1/2 cup apple juice

-1/2 cup plain Greek yogurt

-1 tablespoon honey

-1/2 teaspoon ground cinnamon

Instructions:

1. Put all ingredients in a blender and blend smooth till it is suitable for drinking.

2. Pour into a glass and enjoy.

53. Raspberry-Banana Smoothie:

Ingredients:

-1 cup frozen raspberries

-1/2 cup banana slices

-1/2 cup plain Greek yogurt

-1 tablespoon honey

-1/2 teaspoon ground flaxseed

Instructions:

1. Put all ingredients in a blender and blend smooth till it is suitable for drinking.

2. Pour into a glass and enjoy.

54. Papaya-Mint Smoothie:

Ingredients:

-1 cup papaya chunks

-1/2 cup coconut milk

-1/2 cup plain Greek yogurt

-1 tablespoon honey

-1/2 teaspoon mint extract

Instructions:

1. Put all ingredients in a blender and blend smooth till it is suitable for drinking.

2. Pour into a glass and enjoy.

55. Orange-Ginger Smoothie:

Ingredients:

-1 cup orange juice

-1/2 cup frozen mango chunks

-1/2 cup plain Greek yogurt

-1 tablespoon honey

-1/2 teaspoon ground ginger

Instructions:

1. Put all ingredients in a blender and blend smooth till it is suitable for drinking.

2. Pour into a glass and enjoy.

56. Apple-Blueberry Smoothie:

Ingredients:

-1 cup diced apples

-1/2 cup frozen blueberries

-1/2 cup plain Greek yogurt

-1 tablespoon honey

-1/2 teaspoon ground cinnamon

Instructions:

1. Put all ingredients in a blender and blend smooth till it is suitable for drinking.

2. Pour into a glass and enjoy.

57. Strawberry-Almond Smoothie:

Ingredients:

-1 cup frozen strawberries

-1/2 cup almond milk

-1/2 cup plain Greek yogurt

-1 tablespoon honey

-1/2 teaspoon ground flaxseed

Instructions:

1. Put all ingredients in a blender and blend smooth till it is suitable for drinking.

2. Pour into a glass and enjoy.

58. Pineapple-Coconut Smoothie:

Ingredients:

-1 cup pineapple juice

-1/2 cup frozen pineapple chunks

-1/2 cup coconut milk

-1 tablespoon honey

-1/2 teaspoon ground turmeric

Instructions:

1. Put all ingredients in a blender and blend smooth till it is suitable for drinking.

2. Pour into a glass and enjoy.

59. Peach-Cherry Smoothie:

Ingredients:

-1 cup frozen peaches

-1/2 cup frozen cherries

-1/2 cup plain Greek yogurt

-1 tablespoon honey

-1/2 teaspoon ground nutmeg

Instructions:

1. Put all ingredients in a blender and blend smooth till it is suitable for drinking.

2. Pour into a glass and enjoy.

60. Banana-Cocoa Smoothie:

Ingredients:

-1 cup banana slices

-1/2 cup almond milk

-1/2 cup plain Greek yogurt

-1 tablespoon honey

-1/2 teaspoon cocoa powder

Instructions:

1. Put all ingredients in a blender and blend smooth till it is suitable for drinking.

2. Pour into a glass and enjoy.

Conclusion

In conclusion, Parkinson's Disease is a life-altering condition that can cause a variety of debilitating symptoms. It is important to be aware of the signs and symptoms of the disease and to seek medical advice if you are experiencing any of them.

Treatment options vary, but typically involve a combination of medications, lifestyle changes, and physical or speech therapy. Additionally, there is evidence to suggest that exercise, nutrition, and stress management can help reduce symptoms, slow progression, and improve overall quality of life.

While there is currently no cure for Parkinson's Disease, it is possible to manage the condition and improve overall health with the right knowledge and resources. With the right treatment and support, those living with Parkinson's Disease can enjoy meaningful and fulfilling lives.

The most important thing is to remember that this is a journey, and you do not have to go through it alone. Reach out to your doctor and other healthcare providers, family, and friends for support.

Take advantage of available resources and take care of your physical and mental health. With the right approach, you can take control of your condition and live a full and productive life.

Most importantly, take the time to learn about the condition, speak to your doctor, and explore the available treatment options. With the right attitude and the right resources, you can live a healthy and happy life despite Parkinson's Disease.

Printed in Poland
by Amazon Fulfillment
Poland Sp. z o.o., Wrocław
04 January 2023

100dc3bf-8fec-4ffe-abf2-7476ecce6b04R01